CW00517236

The Super Simple Copycat Recipes

Uncover the Most Selected Restaurant Recipes that Busy People and Beginners can do. Including Steakhouses, Chipotle, Fast Food, Cracker Barrel and much more.

JORDAN BERGSTROM

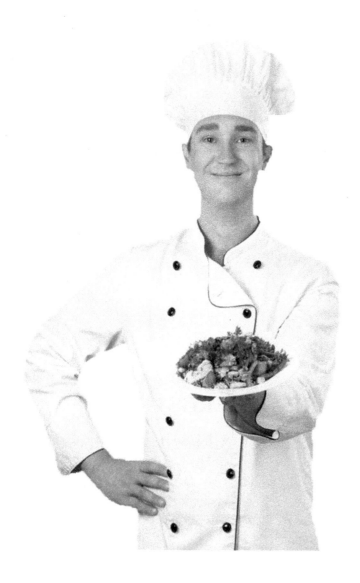

TABLE OF CONTENTS

TABLE OF CONTENTS 3

INTRODUCTION 5

BREAKFAST RECIPES... 7
    DAVE AND BUSTER'S PHILLY STEAK ROLLS 7
    JOE'S CRAB SHACK CRAB DIP 9
    OUTBACK STEAKHOUSE COCONUT SHRIMP 10
    RED LOBSTER CHEDDAR BAY BISCUITS 11
    ARBY'S ROAST BEEF SANDWICH 13
    CALIFORNIA PIZZA KITCHEN WEDGE SALAD 14
    CHILI'S GRILLED CARIBBEAN CHICKEN SALAD 15
    SUBWAY VEGGIE WRAP...17
    STEAK N' SHAKE FRISCO MELT 18
    AUNTIE ANNE'S SOFT PRETZELS 20

APPETIZER RECIPES 22
    CILANTRO LIME DRESSING.. 22
    CRISPY GINGER LIME CHICKEN WINGS 23
    CRISPY BRATWURST WITH GLAZED BRUSSEL SPROUTS............................ 25
    HEALTHY CHICKEN FINGER 28
    PRESSURE COOKER GARLIC "BUTTER" CHICKEN 30
    KETO LEMON BLUEBERRY CHICKEN SALAD 31
    SHEET PAN TACO BOWLS 33
    ROASTED "LOADED" CAULIFLOWER............................. 36
    CREAMY TARRAGON CHICKEN SALAD 38

SOUPS AND BOWL RECIPES.....................................40
    PF CHANG'S SPICY CHICKEN NOODLE SOUP 40
    PF CHANG'S HOT AND SOUR SOUP 43
    LOADED HASH BROWN CASSEROLE 45
    ZUPPA TOSCANA SOUP FROM OLIVE GARDEN........................ 47
    BROCCOLI CHEDDAR SOUP FROM PANERA 49
    TOMATO BASIL SOUP FROM APPLEBEE'S 51
    BAKED POTATO SOUP FROM BENNIGAN'S........................ 53
    CHICKEN SOUP 55

MAIN RECIPES..57
    MELLOW MUSHROOM'S PIZZA HOLY SHIITAKE........................ 57

JIMMY JOHN'S SANDWICH 61
LONG JOHN SILVER'S BATTER-DIPPED FISH 63
OLIVE GARDEN'S STEAK GORGONZOLA ALFREDO 65
CHIPOTLE'S CHIPOTLE PORK CARNITAS 68
KFC FRIED CHICKEN AND COLESLAW 70
LONGHORN'S PARMESAN CRUSTED CHICKEN WITH MASHED POTATOES 73
RED LOBSTER'S SHRIMP SCAMPI WITH CHEDDAR BAY BISCUITS 77
PF CHANG'S SHRIMP DUMPLINGS 81
CHILI'S BBQ BABY BACK RIBS 83
PAPPADEAUX'S CRAWFISH BISQUE 85
WAFFLES HOUSE WAFFLES 88
CRACKER BARREL'S HASH BROWN CASSEROLE 90

PASTA AND PIZZA RECIPES 92

HUMMUS PIZZA WITH VEGGIES 92
RYE CRISPBREAD PIZZA 94
PERFECT PIZZA & PASTRY 95
VERY VEGAN PATRAS PASTA 98
SCRUMPTIOUS SHRIMP PAPPARDELLE PASTA 100

DESSERT RECIPES 102

CINNABON'S CLASSIC CINNAMON ROLLS 102
HOMEMADE ORIGINAL GLAZED DOUGHNUTS FROM KRISPY KREME 104
MRS. FIELDS SNICKERDOODLE COOKIES 107
DIY PUMPKIN SCONES FROM STARBUCKS 109
CLASSIC CHEESECAKE FROM THE CHEESECAKE FACTORY 112
CRACKER BARREL'S DOUBLE FUDGE COCA COLA CHOCOLATE CAKE 115

CONCLUSION 117

INTRODUCTION

Thank you for purchasing this book. Copycat recipes can be so much fun to make, and this book has shown you how.

Family meals have always been a big deal at our house. There's just nothing quite like getting your friends and loved ones together in the dining room to enjoy a tasty, piping hot home cooked meal. I get that some folks love eating out, but for me, you just can't beat a home cooked meal when it comes to cost, health, and really the whole experience! But just like anyone else, I have my favorite foods that I enjoy time to time from restaurants.

There are so many reasons to be a restaurant "copycat" in the kitchen, but when the summer of 2020 hit right as I was finalizing this book, my family suddenly had a whole new reason to appreciate copycat cooking – all the restaurants (and almost everything else) were closed! Even when they reopened, the experience just wasn't the same and the safety risk hardly seemed worth it. Fortunately, with my collection of copycat recipes to rely on, the restaurant in our kitchen never closes and the menu is longer than any restaurant.

Whatever your reasons for copycat cooking, I hope you enjoy my copycat recipes. They are the product of much trial and error and each will allow you to cook a faithful representation of your favorite restaurant dishes at home.

Eating your favorite

restaurant meals at home is just one of the benefits of a copycat recipe. eat at home and save money.

Enjoy your next meal at the best restaurant in town – your dining room!

BREAKFAST RECIPES

Dave and Buster's Philly Steak Rolls

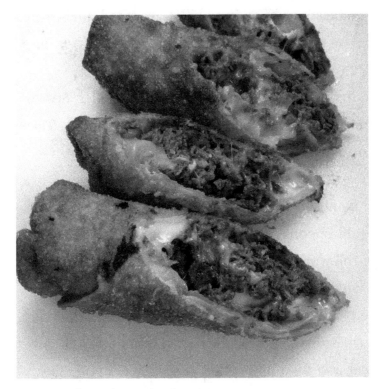

Preparation Time: 6 minutes

Cooking Time: 17 minutes

Serving: 5

Ingredients

- 1 tablespoon vegetable oil
- ½ cup diced onions
- 1 box of Steakums (7 slices)

- Salt and pepper, to taste
- 1 (15-ounce) jar of Cheez Wiz
- 10 egg roll wraps
- 2 cups vegetable oil, for frying

Directions:

1. Cook 1 tablespoon of oil in a skillet over medium heat.
2. Mix in onion and cook, stirring frequently, for 2–3 minutes.
3. Break up Steakums pieces and mix in to skillet. Season salt and pepper to taste; cook and for 7 minutes. Take away from heat and set aside.
4. Situate egg roll wrap on a clean, dry surface with a corner facing you, like a baseball diamond.
5. Put 2 tablespoons of beef and onions onto the center of an egg roll wrap and top with 1–2 tablespoons of Cheese Wiz. Don't overfill your wrapper.
6. Crease corner closest to you over the mixture, then flap side corners over and roll. Seal with water
7. Pre-heat and fill a high-sided pan with 1" of oil. Slowly put the rolls into the oil and cook for 3 to 4 minutes.
8. Strain on paper towels, and serve warm with ketchup.

Nutrition 133 Calories 8.9g Fat 7.2g Protein

Joe's Crab Shack Crab Dip

Preparation Time: 7 minutes

Cooking Time: 4 minutes

Serving: 4

Ingredients

- 1 (5-ounce) can drained crab meat
- 1 (8-ounce) package softened cream cheese
- 3 tablespoons heavy whipping cream
- 2 teaspoons diced onion
- 2 teaspoons diced red pepper
- 2 teaspoons diced green pepper
- 2 teaspoons diced tomato
- 2 teaspoons diced green onion
- 2 teaspoons white wine
- 1 tablespoon Parmesan cheese
- ½ teaspoon Old Bay seasoning
- Dash of Tabasco sauce, to taste

Directions:

1. Using a microwave-safe dish, incorporate all the ingredients.
2. Microwave on medium power for 4 minutes.
3. Pull out from microwave, and stir. Serve with bread.

Nutrition 175 Calories 14g Fat 10g Protein

Outback Steakhouse Coconut Shrimp

Preparation Time: 60 minutes

Cooking Time: 4 minutes

Serving: 2

Ingredients

- 12 jumbo shrimp
- 1 (7-ounce) divided bag shredded coconut
- 2 tablespoons sugar
- ½ teaspoon salt
- 1 cup flour
- 1 cup beer

Directions:

1. Skin and devein the shrimp. Leave the tails on.
2. Mix ½ cup coconut, sugar, salt, flour, and beer well, cover, and chill for a minimum of 60 minutes.
3. Cook oil in a skillet to 350°F.
4. Pour the remainder of the coconut flakes into a shallow bowl. Drench one shrimp simultaneously into the batter, then put the battered shrimp in the coconut.
5. Cook the shrimp for 3 minutes. Strain on paper towels.

Nutrition 307 Calories 17g Fat 11g Protein

Red Lobster Cheddar Bay Biscuits

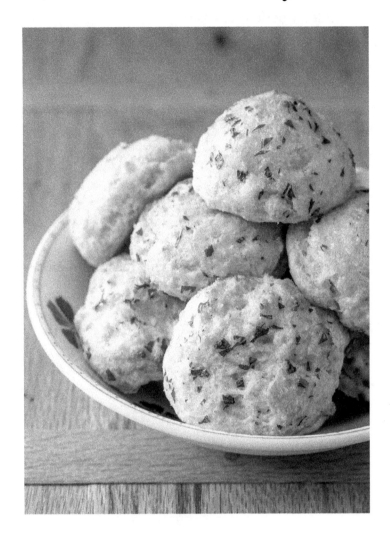

Preparation Time: 21 minutes

Cooking Time: 9 minutes

Serving: 7

Ingredients

- 2 cups Bisquick baking mix

- 2/3 cup milk
- ½ cup shredded Cheddar cheese
- ½ cup melted butter
- ¼ teaspoon garlic powder

Directions:

1. Prep oven to 450°F.
2. Incorporate baking mix, milk, and cheese until a soft dough form.
3. Plop by the spoonful onto an ungreased cooking sheet.
4. Bake for 9 minutes. Blend butter and garlic powder.
5. Coat the butter mixture over warm biscuits before removing from cookie sheet.

Nutrition 122 Calories 7.8g Fat 3.5g Protein

Arby's Roast Beef Sandwich

Preparation Time: 9 minutes

Cooking Time: 2 minutes

Serving: 4

Ingredients

- 1 pound thinly sliced deli roast beef
- 1 can beef broth
- Butter, for brushing
- 4 plain hamburger buns

Direction:

1. Situate the roast beef and broth in a microwave-safe bowl. Heat for 1–2 minutes.
2. Brush a light coating of butter to the inside of the bun and toast lightly in a skillet.
3. Situate the warm roast beef on the bun. Pile as high as you like.
4. Add the barbecue sauce on top of the beef.

Nutrition 320 Calories 13g Fat 20g Protein

California Pizza Kitchen Wedge Salad

Preparation Time: 13 minutes

Cooking Time: 0 minutes

Serving: 2

Ingredients

- 1 head iceberg lettuce
- Blue cheese dressing, to taste
- 2 peeled and chopped hardboiled eggs
- 6 slices chopped cooked bacon
- Blue cheese crumbles, to taste
- ½ cup chopped tomatoes

Directions:

1. Trim off any brown or dark green leaves on the head of lettuce.
2. Remove the inside core by tapping it on a counter top.
3. Slice the head of lettuce in half.
4. Cut the opposite ends so that the lettuce wedge will lay flat.
5. Top the lettuce with blue cheese dressing.
6. Add chopped eggs and bacon.
7. Finish the salad with blue cheese crumbles and tomatoes.

Nutrition 280 Calories 27g Fat 5g Protein

Chili's Grilled Caribbean Chicken Salad

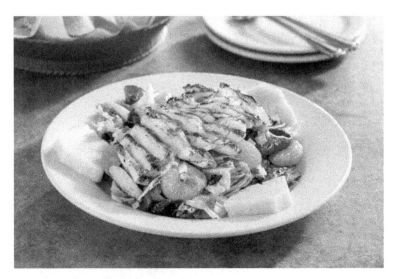

Preparation Time: 3 hours

Cooking Time: 6 minutes

Serving: 4

Ingredients

- 4 boneless, skinless chicken breasts
- ½ cup teriyaki marinade

Honey-Lime Dressing

- ¼ cup Dijon mustard
- ¼ cup honey
- 1½ teaspoons sugar
- 1 tablespoon sesame oil
- 1½ cups apple cider vinegar
- 1½ teaspoons lime juice

Pico De Gallo

- 2 diced tomatoes
- ½ cup diced Spanish onions
- 2 teaspoons chopped jalapeño pepper
- 2 teaspoons minced cilantro
- Pinch of salt

Salad

- 4 cups chopped leaf lettuce
- 4 cups chopped iceberg lettuce
- 1 cup chopped red cabbage
- 1 can drained pineapple chunks
- 4 handfuls of tortilla chips, broken into pieces

Directions:

1. Marinate the chicken in teriyaki marinade for 2 hours in the refrigerator.
2. Incorporate all the ingredients for the dressing in a small bowl and chill for 30 minutes
3. Incorporate all the ingredients for the Pico de Gallo in a small bowl and chill for 30 minutes
4. Prep the grill and grill the chicken breast for 5 minutes on each side or until done. Slice into strips.
5. Throw the lettuce and cabbage in a large salad bowl.
6. Stir in the Pico de Gallo, pineapple, dressing, and tortilla chips.
7. Add the grilled chicken strips. Toss, and serve.

Nutrition 390 Calories 4.5g Fat 34g Protein

Subway Veggie Wrap

Preparation Time: 11 minutes

Cooking Time: 2 minutes

Serving: 1

Ingredients

- ¼ cup refried beans
- 1 slice of cheese of your choice
- 1 whole-wheat tortilla
- ½ cup shredded lettuce
- ½ cup diced tomato
- ¼ cup diced onion
- 4 pickle slices
- 3 diced olives
- 2 teaspoons fat-free Italian salad dressing
- 2 teaspoons honey mustard salad dressing

Directions:

1. Lay out the refried beans and cheese onto the tortilla.
2. Place on a plate and microwave for 30–60 seconds, until the cheese melts.
3. Add the vegetables, pickles, and olives on top of the melted cheese.
4. Drizzle the salad dressings on top of the vegetables.
5. Roll up like a burrito.

Nutrition 130 Calories 3g Fat 12g Protein

Steak n' Shake Frisco Melt

Preparation Time: 12 minutes

Cooking Time: 7 minutes

Serving: 4

Ingredients

- 1 tablespoon ketchup
- 2 tablespoons Thousand Island dressing
- 1-pound ground beef
- 8 slices of bread
- 1 tablespoon butter or margarine
- 2 tablespoons diced onions
- 8 slices American cheese
- 4 slices Swiss cheese
- 4 lettuce leaves
- 4 slices of tomato

Directions:

1. Combine the ketchup and salad dressing. Set aside.
2. Form ground beef into 8 thin patties. Fry or grill the burgers until cooked as desired. Set aside.
3. Lightly toast all 8 slices of bread.
4. To a skillet, add ½ tablespoon of margarine, and cook the onions for 2–3 minutes until softened. Remove the onions and keep aside.

5. Arrange accordingly from bottom to top: bread, American cheese, burger, Swiss cheese, burger, American cheese, onions, salad dressing, and bread.
6. Place sandwich in skillet and toast 1–2 minutes on each side to melt the cheeses.
7. Serve with a lettuce leaf and a tomato slice.

Nutrition 874 Calories 39g Fat 49g Protein

Auntie Anne's Soft Pretzels

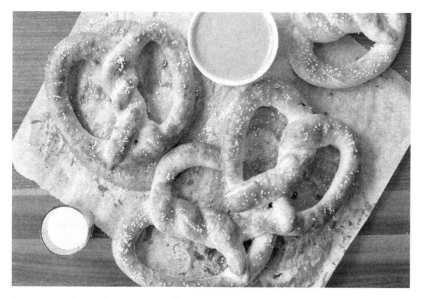

Preparation Time: 32 minutes

Cooking Time: 13 minutes

Serving: 6

Ingredients

- 1½ cups warm water
- 11/8 teaspoons active dry yeast
- 2 tablespoons brown sugar
- 11/8 teaspoons salt
- 1 cup bread flour
- 3 cups regular flour
- 2 cups warm water
- 2 tablespoons baking soda
- Coarse salt, to taste

- 4 tablespoons melted butter

Directions:

1. Preheat oven to 400°F.
2. Add water to a mixing bowl and sprinkle yeast into it. Stir to dissolve.
3. Add the brown sugar and salt. Stir to dissolve.
4. Stir in flour and knead the dough until elastic.
5. Allow the dough rise at least 30 minutes.
6. While rising, prep baking soda water bath with 2 cups water and 2 tablespoons of baking soda
7. Once it risen, poke off bits of dough and roll into a long rope (about ½" or less thick).
8. Drop each pretzel in the soda solution and situate on greased baking sheet. Let the pretzels to rise again. Sprinkle with coarse salt.
9. Bake for 10 minutes, or until golden. Brush with melted butter and serve.

Nutrition 180 Calories 15g Fat 11g Protein

APPETIZER RECIPES

Cilantro Lime Dressing

Preparation time: 8 minutes

Cooking time: 0 minutes

Servings: 4

Ingredients:

- 1 bunch fresh cilantro stems and all*
- 2 large cloves garlic
- 3 tablespoons lime juice
- 6 tablespoons extra virgin olive oil
- 1/2 teaspoon salt
- 1/2 teaspoon red chili flakes
- 1 avocado
- 1-2 tablespoons water (optional)

Direction

1. Incorporate all the ingredients in a blender then blend until smooth. Taste and season with more salt and lime juice as you see fit.

Nutrition: 122 Calories 13g Fat 0.1g Protein

Crispy Ginger Lime Chicken Wings

Preparation time: 16 minutes

Cooking time: 71 minutes

Servings: 10

Ingredient:

- 15 pastured chicken wings
- ½ tablespoon baking powder
- 1 tablespoon fine salt
- 1 tablespoon granulated garlic
- 2 tablespoons avocado oil

For the sauce

- 2 tablespoons avocado oil
- 3 tablespoons coconut amino
- 2 tablespoons apple cider vinegar
- ¼ cup bone broth
- ¼ cup juice from the orange
- zest of orange
- zest of 2 limes
- 6 cloves garlic, zested
- 1-inch nub of ginger, zested
- 1 tablespoon nutritional yeast
- 1 teaspoon turmeric
- 1 teaspoon dried dill weed
- ½ teaspoon garlic powder

- ½ teaspoon ginger powder

Direction

2. Pre-heat oven to 250F. Situate rack over a sheet pan and slightly oil it. Pat your chicken dry.

3. Chop your wings per the instructions above at both joints. Set aside the tips for later use like broth.

4. Put all of the drumettes and vignettes and mix with salt, garlic and baking powder. Stir in the oil and toss again.

5. Arrange all of the chicken pieces up on the rack.

6. Bake at 250F for 35 minutes. Then adjust the oven up to 425F degrees. Bake for extra 42 minutes.

7. Preheat small sauce pot over medium heat. Once it is hot stir in the avocado oil, coconut amino and apple cider vinegar

8. Simmer while you measure out the remaining of the seasoning and zest the fruit.

9. Pour in orange juice and broth to the mix then simmer again until the liquid is decreased by half and lightly coats a spoon.

10. Mix in the zest, yeast and seasonings. Stir until the sauce is like a thick, kind of chunky glaze. Remove from the heat. Go relax, you have some idle time.

11. When done, take them from the oven and toss in a big bowl with the sauce! Serve hot and enjoy.

Nutrition 450 Calories 38g Fat 42g Protein

Crispy Bratwurst with Glazed Brussel Sprouts

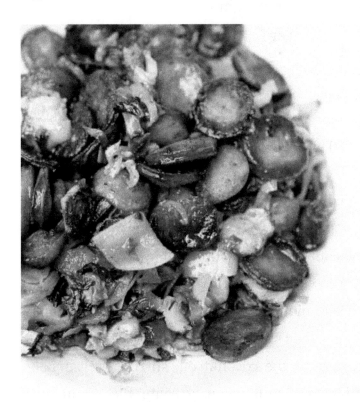

Preparation time: 6 minutes

Cooking time: 17 minutes

Servings: 4

Ingredients:

- 1/4 cup coconut oil, for frying
- 5 fully cooked, pork bratwurst
- 1-pound Brussel sprouts
- 1 large sweet onion
- 3 tablespoons avocado oil

- 1/2 teaspoon fine salt
- 1/2 teaspoon garlic powder
- 3 tablespoons coconut amino
- 1 tablespoon vinegar
- 1 teaspoon fish sauce
- 2 tablespoons pastured gelatin

Direction

1. Preheat two big skillets over medium heat.
2. While they come to temperature cut bratwurst into thin slices, small dice the onion then strip the Brussel sprouts
3. Pour in coconut oil to one skillet and the avocado oil to another. Allow coconut oil heat for extra minute or so. Stir in diced onion to the avocado oil skillet and sauté for 2 minutes then stir in the Brussel sprouts.
4. Fry bratwurst to the coconut oil, stirring occasionally for 9 minutes. Simultaneously sauté the onion and Brussel sprouts. Stir in the salt and garlic powder to the Brussel sprouts.
5. In the small bowl combine the coconut amino, vinegar and fish sauce, then stir in 2 tablespoons of gelatin on top and let it bloom.
6. Reduce the heat on the Brussel sprouts then stir in the gelled sauce mass to the veggie mix. Remove from heat.

7. Put off the heat on the bratwurst skillet. With a slotted spoon to pull out the crispy bratwurst from the coconut oil. Serve.

Nutrition 522 Calories 46g Fat 15g Protein

Healthy Chicken Finger

Preparation time: 17 minutes

Cooking time: 21 minutes

Servings: 4

Ingredients:

- ½ cup coconut flour
- 2 teaspoons poultry seasoning
- ½ tsp. sea salt
- 1 lb. boneless pastured chicken breasts
- ¼ cup avocado oil

Direction

1. Prep oven to 400F.
2. Using shallow bowl or on a plate, mix coconut flour, poultry seasoning, and sea salt.
3. Chop the chicken breast into strips, and brush generously with avocado oil.
4. Soak the oil-coated chicken strips into the coconut flour mixture to coat.
5. Situate finished strips onto a baking sheet one-at-a-time. Once all coated, mist them with a thin coating of oil
6. Bake for 12 minutes, turn over then mist with oil, before returning to the oven for extra 12 minutes.
7. Enjoy with your favorite dip like organic ketchup or homemade paleo mayo!

Nutrition 345 Calories 22g Fat 26g Protein

Pressure Cooker Garlic "Butter" Chicken

Preparation time: 6 minutes

Cooking time: 41 minutes

Servings: 4

Ingredients:

- 4 chicken breasts, whole or chopped
- ¼ cup Coconut Oil
- 1 teaspoon salt (add more to taste)
- 10 cloves garlic, peeled and diced

Direction

1. Stir in chicken breasts to the pressure cooker pot.
2. Add the oil, salt, and diced garlic to the pressure cooker. Adjust pressure cooker on high pressure for 35 minutes. Follow your pressure cooker's directions for releasing the pressure
3. Strip the chicken breast in the pot.

Nutrition 404 Calories 21g Fat 47g Protein

Keto Lemon Blueberry Chicken Salad

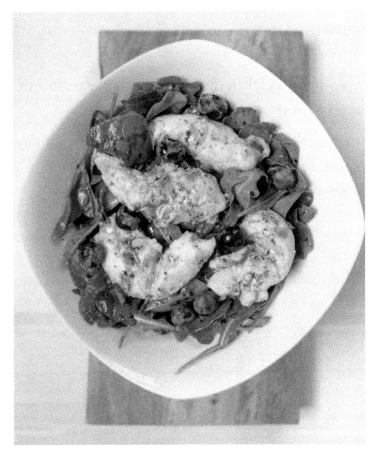

Preparation time: 13 minutes

Cooking time: 11 minutes

Servings: 2

Ingredient:

- 10 blueberries
- 1/4 medium onion
- Large bag of salad leaves
- 2 Tablespoons olive oil

- 2 teaspoons fresh lemon juice
- 1 large chicken breast (1/2 lb.)
- 2 Tablespoons coconut oil to cook in

Direction

1. Cook the diced chicken breast in 2 tablespoons of coconut oil. Sprinkle salt to taste.
2. Throw the cooked chicken with the blueberries, onion slices, salad leaves, olive oil, and lemon juice.

Nutrition: 490 Calories 42g Fat 27g Protein

Sheet Pan Taco Bowls

Preparation time: 12 minutes

Cooking time: 37 minutes

Servings: 2

Ingredients:

For the sheet pan

- 3 tablespoons avocado oil, divided
- 2 cups cauliflower rice, frozen
- 1-pound boneless skinless chicken thighs
- ½ red onion, sliced
- 1 bunch radishes, quartered
- 2 teaspoons pink Himalayan salt
- 1 teaspoon ground ginger
- 1 teaspoon dried parsley
- 1 teaspoon ground turmeric

For the sauce

- 1 bunch cilantro, stems trimmed
- juice of 2 lemons
- 1 tablespoon apple cider or coconut vinegar
- 2 tablespoons coconut manna or coconut butter
- ½ teaspoon fine Himalayan salt
- 1 tablespoon nutritional yeast
- 1 tablespoon coconut amino
- ½ cup avocado oil

To serve

- 1 heart of romaine, shredded
- 1 ripe avocado, sliced

Direction

1. Prep the oven to 400F.
2. Pour 1 tablespoon of avocado oil all over a sheet pan.
3. One on side lay out 2 cups of frozen cauliflower rice.
4. Arrange the chicken thighs so they are lying flat, snug but not overlying.
5. In the space that is left spread the red onion and radishes. Season the salt, getting about 1 teaspoon on the chicken thighs.
6. Stir in remaining seasoning only to the chicken.
7. Sprinkle rest of the oil all over the chicken and rice.
8. Put the sheet pan in the oven and roast for 30 minutes. Then broil for 5 minutes.
9. In the meantime, prepare the rest of the bowls. Shred the lettuce, slice the avocado and make the sauce.
10. Combine the cilantro, nutritional yeast, lemon juice, coconut manna, salt and coconut amino in the blender, and blend on low until almost smooth. Then gradually drizzle in the avocado oil until the sauce is fluid. Take out from the blender and store in the fridge until ready to serve!
11. To assemble your bowls, create a bed of romaine in two bowls. Then scoop the rice on one side, the radishes and onions on another. Find a spot for your avocado. Slice 2

chicken thighs per bowl. Then drizzle sauce over everything.

Nutrition: 391 Calories24g Fat 16g Protein

Roasted "Loaded" Cauliflower

Preparation time: 37 minutes

Cooking time: 31 minutes

Servings: 5

Ingredient:

- 2 heads cauliflower
- 10-12 ounces bacon
- 1 bunch green onions
- 1 cup melting cheese (optional)
- 1 teaspoon sea salt
- several sprigs fresh thyme

Direction

1. Prep oven to 400F. Arrange bacon out on a large baking sheet (preferably a half sheet) Bake for 15-20 minutes.
2. Take the bacon to plate, and set aside. Keep pan with fat.
3. Lay out cauliflower on pan with bacon fat. Sprinkle with sea salt. Mix well with two spoons, so cauliflower is well-coated with fat. Roast cauliflower about 22 minutes.
4. Remove pan from oven. Add green onions' whites and optional cheese. Reduce oven temp to 200F.

5. Put back in oven for 5 minutes. Remove from oven. Situate to serving dish with any pan juices. Top with green onions' greens and fresh thyme. Serve.

Nutrition: 199 Calories 20g Fat 14g Protein

Creamy Tarragon Chicken Salad

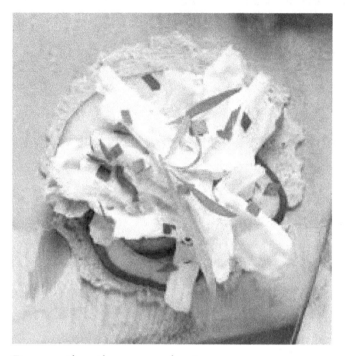

Preparation time: 32 minutes

Cooking time: 0 minutes

Servings: 3

Ingredient:

- 3 cups white chicken meat
- ¼ cup avocado oil
- 2 tbsp sherry vinegar
- 2 medium pears
- ¼ cup red onion
- 2 tbsp fresh tarragon, minced
- 1 tsp sea salt

Direction

1. Situate chopped chicken in a large mixing bowl.
2. Mince the tarragon and add to the bowl, along with the pomegranate seeds if using.
3. Peel and cut the pears, placing 1/2 cup into the mixing bowl.
4. Blend remaining 1 cup of chopped pear, avocado oil, sherry vinegar, and sea salt until thick and smooth.
5. Drizzle the dressing over the chicken and toss around in the bowl until evenly coated then serve over a bed of leafy greens.

Nutrition: 201Calories 24g Fat 16g Protein

SOUPS AND BOWL RECIPES

PF Chang's Spicy Chicken Noodle Soup

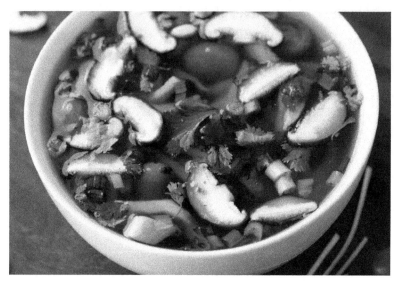

Preparation Time: 10 minutes

Cooking time: 20 minutes

Servings: 6

Ingredients:

- 2 quarts chicken stock
- 1 tablespoon granulated sugar
- 3 tablespoons white vinegar
- 2 cloves garlic, minced
- 1 tablespoon ginger, freshly minced

- ¼ cup soy sauce
- Sriracha sauce to taste
- Red pepper flakes to taste
- 1-pound boneless chicken breast, cut into thin 2–3-inch pieces
- 3 tablespoons cornstarch
- Salt to taste
- 1 cup mushrooms, sliced
- 1 cup grape tomatoes, halved
- 3 green onions, sliced
- 2 tablespoons fresh cilantro, chopped
- ½ pound pasta, cooked to just under package Directions and drained

Directions:

1. Add the chicken stock, sugar, vinegar, garlic, ginger, soy sauce, Sriracha and red pepper flakes to a large saucepan. Boil, then decrease the heat to simmer. Let cook for 5 minutes.

2. Season chicken with salt to taste. In a resealable bag, combine the chicken and the cornstarch. Shake to coat.

3. Add the chicken to the simmering broth a piece at a time. Then add the mushrooms. Continue to cook for another 5 minutes.

4. Stir in the tomatoes, green onions, cilantro, and cooked pasta.

5. Serve with additional cilantro.

Nutrition: 218 Calories 24g Fat 17g Protein

PF Chang's Hot and Sour Soup

Preparation Time: 5 minutes

Cooking time: 5 minutes

Servings: 6

Ingredient:

- 6 oz. chicken breasts, cut into thin strips
- 1-quart chicken stock
- 1 cup soy sauce
- 1 teaspoon white pepper
- 1 (6 oz) can bamboo shoots
- 6 ounces wood ear mushrooms
- ½ cup cornstarch
- ½ cup water
- 2 eggs, beaten
- ½ cup white vinegar
- 6 ounces silken tofu, cut into strips
- Sliced green onions for garnish

Directions:

1. Cook the chicken strips in a hot skillet until cooked through. Set aside.
2. Add the chicken stock, soy sauce, pepper and bamboo shoots to a stockpot and bring to a boil. Stir in the chicken and let cook for about 3–4 minutes.

3. In a small dish, make a slurry with the cornstarch and water. Add a bit at a time to the stockpot until the broth thickens to your desired consistency.
4. Stir in the beaten eggs and cook for about 45 seconds or until the eggs are done.
5. Remove from the heat and add the vinegar and tofu.
6. Garnish with sliced green onions.

Nutrition: 228 Calories 14g Fat 13g Protein

Loaded Hash Brown Casserole

Preparation Time: 15 minutes

Cooking Time: 45 minutes

Servings: 6 to 8

Ingredients:

- 1-pound sausage
- 3 tablespoons chopped red bell pepper
- ½ cup grated American cheese
- ½ cup grated sharp cheddar cheese
- ½ cup grated Monterey Jack cheese
- 1½ cups grated Colby cheese (divided)
- 2 tablespoons butter
- 2 tablespoons flour
- 2 cups milk
- 2 pounds frozen hash browns

Directions:

1. Preheat the oven to 350°F. Cook the sausage in a big skillet at medium high heat while breaking it into bite-sized pieces.
2. Add the red pepper and cook.
3. Drain any grease and set to the side. Melt 2 tablespoons of butter in another skillet. Stir in the flour and let it cook for a minute or so until it starts to brown.

4. Whisk in ¼ cup of the milk and continue to cook and stir until the mixture thickens. Then whisk in the remaining milk and cook a bit longer. I

5. It will thicken up again; when it does, add the cheeses, reserving 1 cup of the Colby cheese for the top of the casserole.

6. In a bowl, combine the hash browns, the cheese sauce you just prepared, and the cooked sausage.

7. Mix together so that everything is combined, then pour into a baking dish and top with the reserved Colby cheese.

8. Cook for about 45 minutes or until the cheese is melted and the casserole is bubbly.

Nutrition: 520 Calories 24g Protein 35g Fat

Zuppa Toscana Soup from Olive Garden

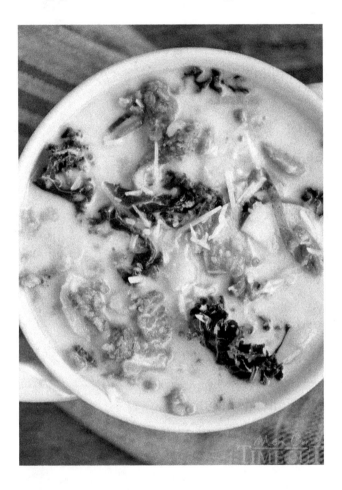

Preparation Time: 18 minutes

Cooking Time: 36 minutes

Servings: 4

Ingredients

Ingredients:

- 16 oz Beef bone broth
- 1 minced cloves garlic

- 1/2 head cauliflower diced
- salt and pepper
- 1/2 lb. mild Italian Sausage
- 1/4 cup heavy whipping cream
- 1 cups spinach
- 2 thick bacon slices
- 1/2 diced small onion

Directions:

1. Cook your bacon (bite-sized) and sausage together with a large soup pot like a Dutch oven until they browned.
2. Add cauliflower, garlic, beef bone broth, and onions into the pot.
3. Cover and cook for about 15 minutes.
4. When the cauliflower is tender, add spinach and heavy cream
5. Cook for an additional 5 minutes.
6. Sprinkle parmesan cheese and a pinch of salt & pepper to taste.
7. Cool before serving.

Nutrition 428 Calories 35g Protein 14g Fat

Broccoli Cheddar Soup from Panera

Preparation Time: 9 minutes

Cooking Time: 39 minutes

Servings: 4

Ingredients

- 2 tbsp melted butter
- 3/4 cup and 2 tbsp broccoli florets, chopped
- 1/2 stalk celery thin slices
- 1/3 cup and 2 tbsp and 1 tsp matchstick-cut carrots
- 2 tbsp melted butter
- 1 cup milk
- salt and black pepper
- 3/4 cup and 1 tbsp and 2 tsp chicken stock
- 1-1/4 cups and 1 tbsp Cheddar cheese
- 1/4 chopped onion
- 2 tbsp flour

Directions:

1. Using medium skillet, cook butter over medium high heat.
2. Place the carrots, onion and salt & pepper and brown until they tender for about 3 to 4 min or more.
3. In a large saucepan, whisk flour and melted butter over medium high heat.
4. If needed, add tbsp of milk to keep the flour from burning. Cook for 3 to 4 minutes.

---

5. Whisk while pouring the milk into the saucepan. Whisk while pouring the milk into the saucepan. Cook until the mixture thickens for approximately 20 minutes.

6. Add the celery, carrot, sauté onion, broccoli and cook for 20 minutes until tender.

7. Place the cheddar cheese in vegetable mixture and stir until the cheese melts. Season with salt and pepper and serve.

Nutrition 298 Calories 13g Protein 10g Fat

Tomato Basil Soup from Applebee's

Preparation Time: 11 minutes

Cooking Time: 39 minutes

Servings: 2

Ingredients

- 1 tsp onion powder
- 4 tbsp erythritol sweetener (granulated)
- 1/2 tsp dried basil
- 28 ounces whole plum tomatoes
- 4 cups of water
- 1/2 cup prepared basil pesto (optional)
- 2 tsp apple cider vinegar
- 3 tsp salt (kosher)
- 2 tbsp butter
- 16 ounces mascarpone cheese
- 1/2 tsp garlic powder

Directions:

1. In a saucepan combine the garlic powder, onion powder, water, canned tomatoes, and salt.
2. Bring to a boil over medium high heat and then simmer for 2 min.
3. Take away from heat, put and puree on the immersion blender or traditional blender until smooth.
4. Put the soup back into the stove, add the mascarpone cheese and butter.

5. Stir over low heat for 2 minutes.

6. Remove from the heat. Stir in the apple cider vinegar, sweetener, pesto, and dried basil.

7. Serve immediately.

Nutrition 262 Calories 5g Protein 24g Fat

Baked Potato Soup from Bennigan's

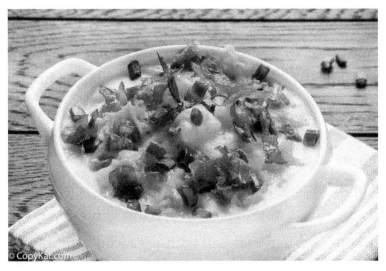

Preparation Time: 13 minutes

Cooking Time: 31 minutes

Servings: 3

Ingredients

- 2.5 c diced and peeled russet potato's
- 1/4 c sliced green onion (greens only) for garnish
- 2 bacon slices
- 1/4 tsp black pepper
- 1/2 c half and half
- 1/2 tsp salt
- 1.5 c shredded cheddar cheese
- 1/4 c flour
- 1/2 c finely diced onion
- 16 oz carton chicken broth

Directions:

1. Using pan, fry bacon over medium heat on each side, until crispy.

2. Remove the bacon from the pan and place them on paper towels. Cook the onion in the remaining fat in the pan where you cooked the bacon.

3. Stir the onion frequently while cooking for 4 - 5 minutes.

4. Add broth, onion, potato, salt & pepper to slow cooker.

5. Cover, set low setting and cook for 6 to 7 hours.

6. Beat flour and half-and-half with wire whisk until well blended in a small bowl, stir into soup.

7. Increase heat setting to high. Cover and cook about 30 minutes longer or until thickened. Stir in 2 cups of cheese until well melted. Spoon into bowls and top with green onion, crumbled bacon, and a bit more cheese.

Nutrition 263 Calories 11g Protein 9g Fat

Chicken Soup

Preparation Time: 14 minutes

Cooking Time: 32 minutes

Servings: 3

Ingredients

- 1 Chicken Breast (cut)
- 1.5 tsp chili powder
- 1/4 chopped onion
- 1/2 cup Monterey Jack cheese, shredded
- 1 tsp Cumin
- 1/2 tbsp avocado oil
- 1 Cups chicken broth (low salt)
- 1 minced garlic clove
- 1/2 tsp xanthan gum
- 1/2 Cup Sauce (Enchilada)
- 1/2 cup cheddar cheese, shredded
- salt and pepper

Direction:

1. Using a big pot, cook avocado oil over medium heat, add in the chicken, garlic, onion and spices. Cook for about 8 minutes.

2. Spill the chicken broth and enchilada sauce. Place and whisk in the xanthan gum and bring it to a boil to thicken. Take out from the heat and season with salt & pepper. Serve in bowls with cheese

Nutrition 284 Calories 20g Protein 18g Fat

MAIN RECIPES

Mellow Mushroom's Pizza Holy Shiitake

Preparation Time: 11 minutes

Cooking Time: 26 minutes

Serving: 3

Ingredients:

- 3 tablespoons truffle oil
- 1 tablespoon butter (melted)
- 3 cups mozzarella cheese
- 4 tablespoons cream cheese
- 1 ½ cups almond flour
- 2 tablespoons baking powder
- 2 tablespoons Swerve sweetener
- 2 egg

Toppings:

- 1 cup mozzarella cheese (shredded)
- 2 cups baby Bella mushrooms (sliced thin)
- ¼ cup oyster mushrooms (chopped)
- ¼ cup shiitake mushrooms (sliced)
- 1 sweet onion (diced)

Aioli Sauce:

- ¾ cup mayo
- 3 garlic cloves (minced)
- 3 tablespoons lemon juice
- ½ teaspoon Himalayan sea salt
- ½ teaspoon black pepper

Direction

1. Set oven to 425 degrees Fahrenheit, then line a baking sheet with parchment paper and set to the side.

2. As the oven preheats, prepare your dough. Take a large, microwave-safe bowl and add in your 3 cups of mozzarella and cream cheese. Situate bowl in the microwave and heat for 1 minute. Stir and heat again for 30 seconds. Keep an eye on the mixture; you just want the cheese to melt and become properly incorporated, not burn.

3. Once the cheese is melted, add in the eggs, almond flour, baking powder, and sweetener. Begin to mix everything together using a fork; it may become easier to just use your hands once a dough begins to form.

4. Situate dough to your prepared baking sheet. Flatten the dough so that it stretches across the sheet or makes a rectangular shape. If the dough is too sticky, run your hands under cool water to help keep the dough from sticking to your fingers.

5. Once the dough is flattened out, use a fork to poke a few holes into the dough. Situate baking sheet into your oven and bake for 8 minutes. After 8 minutes remove your crust from the oven. If there are any bubbles in the crust, use a fork to pop them.

6. Take a small bowl and whisk together your truffle oil and melted butter. Then brush the mixture over the baked crust. Put the crust back to the oven then bake for an additional 10 minutes.

7. As the crust continues to bake, prepare your toppings. Place a saucepan on your stove and turn the heat to medium. Add in your onions and sauté them until they turn a golden-brown color. Add your baby Bella, shiitake, and oyster mushrooms to the pot. Allow the mushrooms to cook for 3 minutes, then turn off the heat.

8. Once your crust has turned a nice golden-brown color, remove it from the oven. Sprinkle your mozzarella cheese over the top then pour the mushroom mixture over the cheese. Return the pizza to the oven and bake for 3 more minutes or until the cheese has melted. Pull out the pizza from the oven and allow it to cool slightly.

9. As the pizza cools, prepare your aioli sauce. Take a small mixing bowl and stir together the mayonnaise, minced garlic cloves, lemon juice, sea salt, and black

pepper. Drizzle your sauce over the pizza then cut into 16 equal squares and serve.

Nutrition 219 Calories 21g Fat 6g Protein

Jimmy John's Sandwich

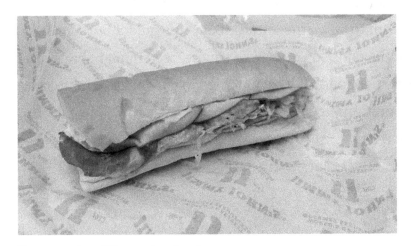

Preparation Time: 6 minutes

Cooking time: 0 minute

Serving: 2

Ingredients:

- 2 slices turkey breast
- 1 slice provolone cheese
- 2 large iceberg lettuce leaves
- 1 tomato (sliced)
- 1 cucumber (sliced)
- ½ avocado (sliced)
- 1 teaspoon mayonnaise
- 1 teaspoon yellow mustard

Directions:

1. Place your lettuce leaves flat on a plate. Then, layer a slice of your turkey, then provolone, and another slice of turkey. Next, add 3 tomato slices, 5 cucumber slices,

and your avocado slices. Top with mayonnaise and mustard.

2. Begin to wrap the lettuce like you would a burrito. Fold in the ends so you have a square/rectangular shape, the start at one of the unfolded ends and begin to roll everything together. Secure with a toothpick or pick up and enjoy!

Nutrition 422 Calories 32g Fat 18g Protein

Long John Silver's Batter-Dipped Fish

Preparation Time: 7 minutes

Cooking Time: 11 minutes

Serving: 4

Ingredients:

- 4 cups vegetable oil (for frying)
- 2 pounds cod (cut into three-inch pieces)
- 16 ounces club soda
- ¼ cup ground flaxseed
- 2 cups almond flour
- ½ teaspoon paprika
- ½ teaspoon onion salt
- ½ teaspoon baking soda
- ½ teaspoon baking powder
- 1 teaspoon Himalayan sea salt
- ¼ teaspoon black pepper

Directions:

1. First, take a deep-frying pan and fill it with the 4 cups of oil. Set heat to medium to pre-heat the oil.

2. As the oil heats, combine the almond flour and ground flaxseed with the paprika, onion salt, baking soda, baking powder, sea salt, and black pepper into a medium-sized mixing bowl. Whisk everything together so it is well incorporated, then add the club soda. Whisk again until the batter has a foamy consistency.

3. Take your cod pieces and dip them into your batter. Ensure that each piece is coated completely then carefully place them into the preheated oil. Do not overcrowd your pan or your fish will not cook evenly. If needed, fry in two batches. Allow the fish to fry for 5 minutes. The fish should have a nice golden color and will begin to float on the oil when done.

4. Remove the fish from the oil using a slotted spoon and transfer them to a plate lined with paper towels to catch the excess oil.

5. Serve with your favorite side!

Nutrition 559 Calories 43g Fat 37g Protein

Olive Garden's Steak Gorgonzola Alfredo

Preparation Time: 42 minutes

Cooking Time: 23 minutes

Serving: 4

Ingredients:

- 1 pound of steak medallions
- 1 tablespoon balsamic vinegar
- ½ teaspoon Himalayan sea salt
- ½ teaspoon black pepper
- 5 zucchinis
- 4 ounces gorgonzola crumbles
- ¼ cup sun-dried tomatoes

For the Sauce

- 2 cups heavy cream
- 1 stick of unsalted butter
- 1 cup parmesan cheese
- 2 cups spinach
- ¼ teaspoon nutmeg
- ¼ teaspoon Himalayan sea salt
- ¼ teaspoon black pepper

Directions:

1. Begin by marinating your steaks. First, sprinkle them with the Himalayan sea salt and black pepper, then

place them in a sealable bag. Add the balsamic vinegar to the bag and seal. Place the steaks in your refrigerator for at least 30 minutes before cooking

2. As the steaks marinate, place a large pot of water on your stovetop and turn the heat to medium high. Then take a spiralizer and create your "fettuccine noodles" using the zucchini. When done, add them to your boiling pot of water for 3 minutes. Then, drain the water and transfer your zucchini noodles to a plate lined with a paper towel, so the excess water can drain off.

3. Get skillet and place it on your stove. Set the heat to medium and allow it to heat up. Remove your steak medallions and place them into the hot skillet. Let them to cook on each side for about five minutes. The thickness of the steak will determine how long you need to cook the steaks. Steaks that are a little over two inches should reach a medium cook in 5 minutes per side.

4. Once the steaks have reached your desired cook time, remove them from the skillet and place them on a plate, then cover them with aluminum foil to rest. Keep in mind your steaks will still continue to cook even though you have removed them from the skillet.

5. As the steaks rest, you want to make your sauce. Place a medium-sized saucepan on your stove and turn the heat

to medium. Add in the butter and heavy cream. Once the butter has begun to melt, add in your spinach. Allow the spinach to cook down; this should only take about 5 minutes. Once the spinach has wilted, add in the parmesan cheese, sea salt, and black pepper. Stir, decrease heat to medium low and allow the sauce to thicken slightly for about 5 minutes.

6. Once the sauce is done, turn off the heat. Transfer your zucchini noodles to a large bowl and pour the sauce over top (leave a little sauce in the saucepan to top your steaks with). Toss the zucchini noodles with the sauce so that everything gets nicely coated. Add in the gorgonzola cheese, but reserve some to top your steaks with during plating. Toss everything one more time.

7. Now it is time to assemble the plate! Place a small portion of the zucchini noodles on your dinner plate, place a steak medallion on top of the noodles, and top with the dried tomatoes, gorgonzola crumbles, and a little drizzle of your leftover sauce.

Nutrition 413 Calories 28g Fat30g Protein

Chipotle's Chipotle Pork Carnitas

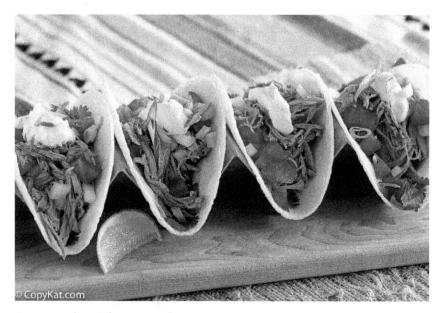

Preparation Time: 7 minutes

Cooking Time: 4 hours

Serving: 4

Ingredients:

- 1 cup water
- 2 tablespoons avocado oil
- 4 pounds pork roast
- 1 teaspoon thyme
- 2 teaspoon juniper berries
- 1 teaspoon Himalayan sea salt
- ½ teaspoon black pepper

Directions:

1. Set oven to 300 degrees Fahrenheit.

2. Next, take a Dutch oven pot, place it on your stove, and turn the heat to medium. Add the avocado oil to the pot.

3. As the pot heats, take your pork roast and sprinkle it with the sea salt. Then place the roast into the Dutch oven pot and brown the sides for a minute on each side.

4. Turn the heat off on the stove once the roast has browned. Add the water, thyme, juniper berries, and black pepper to the pot, then cover. Place the pot into your preheated oven and allow the roast to cook for 3 ½ hours. Flip the roast every 30 minutes so that the flavors really penetrate into all areas of the meat.

5. Remove the roast from the oven after 3 ½ hours (keep the oven turned on), allow it to rest for 10 minutes, then use two forks to pull the meat apart. Once all the meat has been pulled, place the pot back into the oven for 30 minutes.

6. Remove the pot and enjoy!

Nutrition 317 Calories 15g Fat 43g Protein

KFC Fried Chicken and Coleslaw

Preparation Time: 4 hours

Cooking Time: 22 minutes

Serving: 3

Ingredients:

- 8 cups olive oil
- 2 pounds chicken drumsticks
- 1 ½ cups whey protein powder
- 4 tablespoons white vinegar
- 3 tablespoons heavy cream
- 2 cups almond milk (unsweetened)
- 2 eggs

Seasoning:

- 1 teaspoon celery salt
- 1 teaspoon ginger powder
- 2 teaspoon garlic salt
- 4 teaspoons paprika
- ¼ teaspoon oregano (dried)
- ½ teaspoon thyme (dried)
- 1 teaspoon mustard powder
- 1 tablespoon black pepper
- 1 teaspoon Himalayan sea salt

For the Coleslaw:

- ¾ cup mayonnaise

- 2 cup carrots (shredded)
- 3 cups white cabbage (shredded)
- 1 cup purple cabbage (shredded)
- ¼ cup white wine vinegar
- ½ teaspoon garlic powder
- ¼ teaspoon celery salt
- 1/3 cup sour cream
- ½ teaspoon mustard
- ½ teaspoon Himalayan sea salt

Directions:

1. First, prepare your seasoning by mixing all ingredients under the seasoning section in the ingredient list into a small bowl. Divide the mixture in half and set to the side.

2. Next, take a large bowl and pour in the almond milk, white vinegar, heavy cream, and eggs. Whisk everything together thoroughly. Then add in half of the seasoning mixture and whisk until you have a nice smooth mixture.

3. Take your chicken drumsticks and place them into a sealable plastic bag or a large airtight container. Pour in the almond milk mixture and ensure that all the chicken is well coated. Seal the bag or place the lid on your container and place it into your refrigerator for at least 4 hours.

4. When your chicken is done marinating, take a large skillet and pour in the olive oil. Set heat to medium high and allow the oil to become hot.

5. Once the oil is at the appropriate temperature, take a rimmed plate and spread out the rest of the seasoning onto it. Take your marinated chicken and coat each piece with the seasoning mixture, then carefully place the chicken into the hot oil. Allow each drumstick to cook for 20 minutes; the internal temperature should be 165 degrees Fahrenheit. When your chicken is done, remove it from the pan and place it on a plate lined with paper towels to catch the excess grease.

6. Serve with a side of coleslaw.

For the Coleslaw:

1. In a big salad bowl, mix shredded carrots and white and purple cabbage. Toss everything together and set to the side.

2. Take a smaller mixing bowl and combine the mayonnaise, white wine vinegar, celery salt, sour cream, mustard, and sea salt. Whisk so that everything is thoroughly mixed.

3. Pour your mayonnaise mixture over your cabbage mixture and toss until everything is well coated. Place the bowl, covered, into your refrigerator and chill for 30 minutes before serving.

Nutrition 376 Calories 29g Fat 17g Protein

Longhorn's Parmesan Crusted Chicken with Mashed Potatoes

Preparation Time: 53 minutes

Cooking Time: 21 minutes

Serving: 3

Ingredients:

- 2 tablespoons avocado oil
- 4 chicken breasts (boneless, skinless)
- 1 cup panko breadcrumbs
- ¾ cup parmesan cheese
- ¾ cup provolone cheese
- ¼ cup heavy cream
- 1 teaspoon onion powder
- 2 teaspoons garlic powder
- 1 teaspoon dill (dried)
- 1 teaspoon parsley (dried)
- 1 teaspoon chives (dried)
- 2 teaspoon Himalayan sea salt
- 2 teaspoon black pepper

For the Marinade:

- ½ cup avocado oil
- 2 garlic cloves (minced)
- 1 teaspoon lemon juice
- 3 tablespoons Worcestershire sauce

- 1 teaspoon white vinegar
- ½ teaspoon black pepper
- ½ cup keto ranch dressing
- Cauliflower Rive
- 2 tablespoons olive oil
- 1 cauliflower head (should yield 4 cups of "rice")
- ½ teaspoon Himalayan sea salt
- ¼ teaspoon black pepper

Directions:

1. First, you want to prepare your chicken. Take each breast and use a meat tenderizer mallet. I also prefer the old-fashioned way of just using a rolling pin and pounding each breast so they are about ¾" thick. Then season each breast with ½ teaspoon of sea salt and black pepper. Next, take a small mixing bowl to whisk up your marinade. Combine the ½ cup avocado oil, minced garlic cloves, lemon juice, Worcestershire sauce, white vinegar, and keto-friendly ranch dressing. Whisk everything thoroughly. Place your chicken breast into a sealable plastic bag and pour the marinade sauce into the bag. Seal the bag then shake to ensure all the breasts are nicely coated. Place the bag into your refrigerator for at least 30 minutes.

2. Once the chicken has marinated, place a large skillet on your stovetop with 2 tablespoons of avocado oil in it. Set heat to medium to allow the oil to heat up. Remove

your chicken from the bag and carefully place them into the hot skillet. Cook both sides of the chicken for 10 minutes then transfer them to a baking dish to rest.

3. As your chicken is resting, preheat your oven to 450 degrees Fahrenheit.

4. Next, you need a small microwave-safe mixing bowl and add your heavy cream, parmesan cheese, provolone cheese, onion powder, dill, parsley, and chives. Mix everything together and then place the bowl into your microwave and heat for 30 seconds. Remove and stir, microwave for another 15 seconds, stir, and repeat until you have a smooth, creamy mixture. Pour this mixture over your chicken breasts and place your baking dish into the oven. Allow the chicken to bake for 5 minutes.

5. While the chicken bakes, take a small bowl and combine the panko breadcrumbs and garlic powder. Stir everything together. Once the chicken has been in the oven for 5 minutes, remove the dish and sprinkle the breadcrumbs over top. Place the dish back in the oven and bake for another 5 minutes or until the breadcrumbs have turned a lovely golden-brown color.

6. Remove from the oven and serve with cauliflower rice

To Make Cauliflower Rice:

1. Begin by creating your rice. You can do this by chopping the cauliflower into pieces and then adding them to a food processor and pulsing, or you can use a grater to

grate the cauliflower into small rice bits. Once you have rice, sprinkle your sea salt and black pepper over top and gently mix everything together.

2. Take a large skillet and place it on your stove with the olive oil in it. Turn the heat to medium high and allow the oil to get hot.

3. Place your riced cauliflower into the skillet and cook for 5 minutes, stirring occasionally. The cauliflower should be soft and not mushy. Then turn off the heat and enjoy!

Nutrition 557Calories 42g Fat 31g Protein

Red Lobster's Shrimp Scampi with Cheddar Bay Biscuits

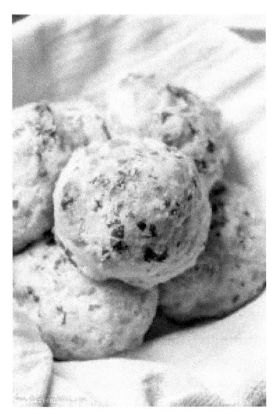

Preparation Time: 13 minutes

Cooking Time: 27 minutes

Serving: 3

Ingredients:

For the Scampi

- 1 ¼ pounds shrimp (peeled, tail removed, deveined)
- 2 garlic cloves (minced)
- 2 scallions (sliced)

- 4 tablespoons butter (unsalted)
- 1/3 cup parmesan cheese (shredded)
- ¼ cup lemon juice
- ¼ cup chardonnay
- ¼ cup parsley (chopped)
- ¼ teaspoon red pepper flakes

For the Biscuits

- 1 ½ cups almond flour
- 2 eggs
- 1 ½ teaspoons garlic powder (separated into 1 and then ½ teaspoon)
- 1 tablespoon baking powder
- ½ cup cheddar cheese (shredded)
- ½ cup sour cream
- 6 tablespoons butter (unsalted, melted, separated into 4 and then 2 tablespoons)
- 1 tablespoon parsley (minced)
- ½ teaspoon Himalayan sea salt

Directions:

1. Situate big skillet on your stove and turn the heat to medium with the butter in it. Allow the skillet to heat up for a few minutes until the butter has melted then add the garlic. Cook the garlic for 1 minute so that it becomes a light golden color.

2. Cook shrimp in the skillet. Let them cook for 3 minutes. Sprinkle the red pepper flake over the shrimp, flip, and cook for another 3 minutes.

3. Once the shrimp have turned a pink color, pour in the lemon juice and chardonnay. Allow everything to simmer for 2 minutes then turn off the heat.

4. Add the scallion and parsley to the skillet. Stir everything together and top with the parmesan cheese.

5. Serve over top of your favorite vegetable noodles like zucchini or spaghetti squash.

6. To make the Biscuits:

7. Set oven to 450 degrees Fahrenheit, then grease a muffin pan with oil and set to the side.

8. In a large mixing bowl, add your almond flour, 1 teaspoon garlic, baking powder, and salt. Use a fork to mix everything together, set to the side.

9. In a small bowl, crack your eggs then pour in four tablespoons of the melted butter and the sour cream. Beat the eggs and sour cream until well incorporated, then add to your flour mixture. Stir your ingredients together until you have a smooth batter, then fold in your cheddar cheese.

10. Take your muffin pan and fill each section with the batter. Place your pan into the oven and bake for 10 minutes.

11. As the biscuits bake, take a small bowl and add the remaining 2 tablespoons of butter and ½ teaspoon of garlic powder. Stir together until the garlic powder has dissolved then add your parsley. Once the biscuits have been removed from the oven, brush each one with your butter and parsley mixture then serve warm.

Nutrition 591 Calories 39g Fat 45g Protein

PF Chang's Shrimp Dumplings

Preparation Time: 20 minutes

Cooking Time: 10 minutes

Servings: 4-6

Ingredients:

- 1-pound medium shrimp, peeled, deveined, washed and dried, divided
- 2 tablespoons carrot, finely minced
- 2 tablespoons green onion, finely minced
- 1 teaspoon ginger, freshly minced
- 2 tablespoons oyster sauce
- ¼ teaspoon sesame oil
- 1 package wonton wrappers

Sauce

- 1 cup soy sauce
- 2 tablespoons white vinegar
- ½ teaspoon chili paste
- 2 tablespoons granulated sugar
- ½ teaspoon ginger, freshly minced
- Sesame oil to taste
- 1 cup water
- 1 tablespoon cilantro leaves

Directions:

1. Using a food processor, finely mince ½ pound of the shrimp.

2. Dice the other ½ pound of shrimp.

3. In a mixing bowl, combine both the minced and diced shrimp with the remaining ingredients.

4. Spoon about 1 teaspoon of the mixture into each wonton wrapper. Wet the edges of the wrapper with your finger, then fold up and seal tightly.

5. Cover and chill for 60 minutes.

6. Incorporate all the ingredients for the sauce and stir until well combined.

7. When ready to serve, boil water in a saucepan and cover with a steamer. You may want to lightly oil the steamer to keep the dumplings from sticking. Steam the dumplings for 7–10 minutes.

8. Serve with sauce.

Nutrition 264 Calories 7.5g Fat 43g Protein

Chili's BBQ Baby Back Ribs

Preparation Time: 11 minutes

Cooking Time: 3 hours

Serving: 5

Ingredients:

- 2 tablespoons avocado oil (divided)
- 2 racks baby back ribs (remove membrane)
- ½ cup BBQ sauce (low carb)
- 1 teaspoon paprika
- 1 teaspoon garlic powder
- 1 teaspoon onion powder
- 1 teaspoon ground mustard
- ½ teaspoon cinnamon
- ½ teaspoon celery salt
- ½ teaspoon cayenne pepper
- 1 teaspoon Himalayan sea salt
- 1 teaspoon black pepper

Directions:

1. First, turn your oven to 275 degrees Fahrenheit.
2. Next, prepare your seasoning rub by combining the paprika, garlic powder, onion powder, ground mustard, cinnamon, celery salt, cayenne pepper, sea salt, and black pepper in a small mixing bowl. Use a fork to stir everything together.

3. Take your racks of ribs and generously rub your seasoning mix all over them. Leave a little of the seasoning mix aside for later.

4. Place your ribs on a rimmed baking sheet, cover, and seal with aluminum foil. Place the baking sheet into your preheated oven and allow the ribs to cook for 2 ½ hours. You'll be tempted to check on them because the smell will fill your home, but resist the urge to peek at them.

5. After 2 ½ hours, take the baking sheet from the oven and uncover. Sprinkle the leftover seasoning mix over top and pour the BBQ sauce over top. Return the baking sheet into the oven for another 30 minutes.

6. The ribs should be a rich dark-red color when done. After removing them from the oven. allow them to rest for 10 minutes before serving.

Nutrition 483 Calories 41g Fat24g Protein

Pappadeaux's Crawfish Bisque

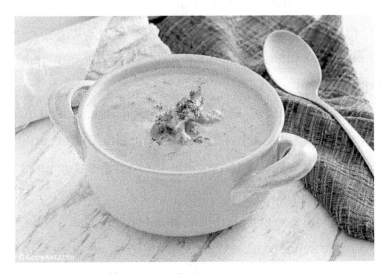

Preparation Time: 17 minutes

Cooking Time: 2 hours

Serving: 3

Ingredients:

- 4 cups water
- 1 tablespoon olive oil
- 1 ½ pounds of crawfish
- ¼ cup tomatoes (chopped)
- ¼ cup onions (chopped)
- ¼ cup green bell pepper (chopped)
- 1 ½ cups heavy cream
- ½ tablespoon tomato paste
- ½ teaspoon paprika
- ¼ teaspoon cayenne pepper

Directions:

1. Take a large pot filled with water and place it on your stove. Turn the heat to high to bring to a boil. Once the water is boiling, add your crawfish and boil for 15 minutes. Then turn off the heat and allow the crawfish to cool for 15 minutes.

2. Take the crawfish and separate the tail meat, set the shells and heads in a bowl to use for the stock later, and put the meat in a bowl to store in the refrigerator until you are ready for it.

3. When you have separated the meat from the shells, place a large saucepan on your stove with the olive oil in it and turn the heat to medium heat. Add the heads and shells from the crawfish to the saucepan along with the cayenne pepper and paprika. Allow everything to sauté over medium heat for 5 minutes. Then, add the water and bring everything to a boil. Once the liquids are boiling, lower the heat to medium low and simmer for 30 minutes.

4. After 30 minutes, strain the liquid from the pan into a medium-sized bowl using a cheesecloth. Discard the shells and heads, then pour the liquid back into the saucepan. Set heat to medium low and add in the tomato paste, heavy cream, chopped tomatoes, onions, and green bell peppers. Allow the vegetables to simmer for 1 hour then add in the crawfish meat. Simmer everything for another 15 minutes. Serve

Nutrition 275 Calories 18g Fat25g Protein

Waffles House Waffles

Preparation Time: 17 minutes

Cooking Time: 24 minutes

Serving: 3

Ingredients:

- 5 eggs (separated)
- 3 tablespoons heavy cream
- ½ cup butter
- 4 tablespoons coconut flour
- 4 tablespoon erythritol (granulated)
- 1 teaspoon baking powder
- 2 teaspoon vanilla extract

Directions:

1. First, take a large mixing bowl and add in your egg yolks, coconut flour, granulated erythritol, and baking powder. Whisk everything together then mix in your melted butter. Continue to whisk until you have a smooth consistency, then add in the heavy cream and vanilla extract. Whisk again until everything is well incorporated, set to the side.

2. Take a medium-sized mixing bowl and add in your egg whites. Take a hand mixer and beat the egg whites until they become nice and firm. When the whites are able to hold a peak, they are ready.

3. Use a large spoon to scoop some of the egg whites into the egg yolk mixture. Use a baking spatula to fold in egg whites, then spoon in more; fold and continue until all the egg whites have been combined with the egg yolks. Don't overmix, you want the mixture to maintain some of the light fluffiness from the egg whites.

4. Take your waffle iron and turn it on. Use a spoon to fill the waffle maker and cook for about 5 minutes (cook time may vary depending on your model of waffle maker, double-check the user manual for approximate cook time). When the waffle is golden brown, it is done. Continues until all your waffle batter has been used.

Nutrition 311 Calories 28g Fat 8g Protein

Cracker Barrel's Hash Brown Casserole

Preparation Time: 7 minutes

Cooking Time: 1 hour

Serving: 4

Ingredients:

- 1 ½ cups cauliflower (shredded)
- ½ cup sour cream
- ½ cup cheddar cheese (shredded, divided)
- ½ cup Monterey jack cheese (shredded, divided)
- ¼ cup mayonnaise
- ½ tablespoon onion powder
- ½ tablespoon bouillon powder
- ½ teaspoon Himalayan sea salt
- ½ teaspoon black pepper

Direction:

1. Set oven to 350F.
2. As the oven preheats, take a large mixing bowl and add ½ cup of the cheddar cheese and ½ cup of the Monterey Jack cheese. Next, add the cauliflower, sour cream, mayonnaise, onion powder, bouillon powder, sea salt, and black pepper. Use a baking spatula to gently mix everything together.
3. Pour the mixture into a greased 8x8 baking dish. Top with the remaining cheddar and Monterey Jack cheese, then place the baking dish into the oven and bake for 1

hour. The dish is done when the top is an irresistible golden-brown color.

4. Pull out from the oven and divide into four equal portions.

Nutrition 242 Calories 20g Fat 9g Protein

PASTA AND PIZZA RECIPES

Hummus Pizza with Veggies

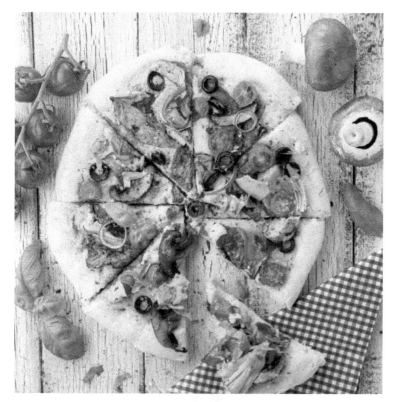

Preparation Time: 15 Minutes

Cooking Time: 15 Minutes

Servings: 4

Ingredients:

- 1 (10 ounces can refrigerated whole-wheat pizza crust dough
- 1 cup broccoli florets
- 1 cup hummus spread
- 2 cups shredded Cheddar cheese
- 1½ cups sliced bell pepper, any color

Directions:

1. Preheat the oven to 475°F.
2. Roll out pizza crust then place on a baking sheet or pizza pan.
3. Spread a thin coating of hummus over the pizza crust.
4. Arrange broccoli and peppers over the hummus, and top with shredded cheese.
5. Bake for 10-15 minutes, until the pizza crust is golden brown and cheese is melted in the center. Slice and serve.

Nutrition: Calories: 251 Protein: 13 g Fat: 12 g Carbs: 122 g

Rye Crispbread Pizza

Preparation Time: 10 Minutes

Cooking Time: 7 Minutes

Servings: 2

Ingredients:

- 8 slices rye crispbread
- 8 cherry tomatoes
- 8 mini mozzarellas
- 4 ounces pizza cheese, grated
- 1 Tbsp. olive oil
- 2 Tbsp. basil, chopped

Directions:

1. Preheat oven to 400°F.
2. Top crispbreads with olive oil, cheese, tomatoes, and basil.
3. Bake for 7 minutes or until the color has changed.

Nutrition: Calories: 110 Protein: 4 g Fat: 4 g Carbs: 6 g

Perfect Pizza & Pastry

Preparation Time: 35 Minutes

Cooking Time: 15 Minutes

Servings: 10

Ingredients:

- 2-tsp honey
- ¼-oz. active dry yeast
- 1¼-cups warm water (about 120 °F)
- 2-tbsp olive oil
- 1-tsp sea salt
- 3-cups whole grain flour + ¼-cup, as needed for rolling
- 1-cup pesto sauce (refer to Perky Pesto recipe)
- 1-cup artichoke hearts
- 1-cup wilted spinach leaves
- 1-cup sun-dried tomato
- ½-cup Kalamata olives
- 4-oz. feta cheese
- 4-oz. mixed cheese of equal parts low-fat mozzarella, asiago, and provolone
- Olive oil
- Bell pepper
- Chicken breast, strips
- Fresh basil
- Pine nuts

Directions:

1. Preheat your oven to 350 °F.

2. Combine the honey and yeast with the warm water in your food processor with a dough attachment. Blend the mixture until fully combined. Allow the combination to rest for 5 minutes to ensure the activity of the yeast through the appearance of bubbles on the surface.

3. Pour in the olive oil. Add the salt, and blend for half a minute. Add gradually 3 cups of flour, about half a cup at a time, blending for a couple of minutes between each addition.

4. Let your processor knead the mixture for 10 minutes until smooth and elastic, sprinkling it with flour whenever necessary to prevent the dough from sticking to the processor bowl's surfaces.

5. Take the dough from the bowl. Let it stand for 15 minutes, covered with a moist, warm towel.

6. By means of a rolling pin, roll out the dough to a half-inch thickness, dusting it with flour as needed. Poke holes indiscriminately on the dough using a fork to prevent crust bubbling.

7. Place the perforated, rolled dough on a pizza stone or baking sheet. Bake for 5 minutes.

8. Lightly brush the baked pizza shell with olive oil.

9. Pour over the pesto sauce and spread thoroughly over the pizza shell's surface, leaving out a half-inch space around its edge as the crust.

10. Top the pizza with artichoke hearts, wilted spinach leaves, sun-dried tomatoes, and olives. (Top with more add-ons, as desired.) Cover the top with the cheese.

11. Place the pizza on the oven rack. Bake for 10 minutes until the cheese is bubbling and melting from the center to the edge. Let the pizza cool for 5 minutes beforehand slicing.

Nutrition: Calories: 242 Protein: 14 g Fat: 15 g Carbs: 16 g

Very Vegan Patras Pasta

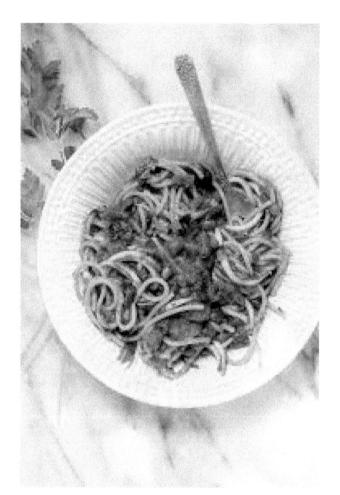

Preparation Time: 5 Minutes

Cooking Time: 10 Minutes

Servings: 6

Ingredients:

- 4-quarts salted water
- 10-oz. gluten-free and whole-grain pasta
- 5-cloves garlic, minced

- 1-cup hummus
- Salt and pepper
- 1/3-cup water
- ½-cup walnuts
- ½-cup olives
- 2-tbsp dried cranberries (optional)

Directions:

1. Bring the salted water to a boil for cooking the pasta.
2. In the meantime, prepare for the hummus sauce. Combine the garlic, hummus, salt, and pepper with water in a mixing bowl. Add the walnuts, olive, and dried cranberries, if desired. Set aside.
3. In the steam shower. Cook the pasta following the manufacturer's specifications until attaining an al dente texture. Drain the pasta.
4. Transfer the pasta to a large bowl and combine with the sauce.

Nutrition: Calories: 329 Protein: 12 g Fat: 13 g Carbs: 43 g

Scrumptious Shrimp Pappardelle Pasta

Preparation Time: 10 Minutes

Cooking Time: 20 Minutes

Servings: 4

Ingredients:

- 3-quarts salted water
- 1-lb. jumbo shrimp, peeled and deveined
- ½-tsp kosher salt
- ¼-tsp black pepper, freshly grated
- 3-tbsp olive oil (divided)
- 2-cups zucchini, cut diagonally to 1/8-inch-thick slices
- 1-cup grape tomatoes halved
- 1/8-tsp. red pepper flakes
- 2-cloves garlic, minced
- 1 tsp. zest of 1-pc lemon
- 2-tbsp lemon juice
- 1-tbsp Italian parsley, chopped
- 8-oz. fresh pappardelle pasta

Directions:

1. Bring the salted water to a boil for cooking the pasta.
2. In the meantime, prepare for the shrimp. Combine the shrimp plus salt and pepper. Set aside.
3. Heat a tablespoon of oil in a large sauté pan placed over medium heat. Add the zucchini slices and sauté for 4 minutes until they are tender.

4. Add the grape tomatoes and sauté for 2 minutes until they just start to soften. Stir in the salt to combine with the vegetables. Transfer the cooked vegetables to a medium-sized bowl. Set aside.

5. In the same sauté pan, pour in the remaining oil. Switch the heat to medium-low. Add the red pepper flakes and garlic. Cook for 2 minutes, stirring regularly so that the garlic will not burn.

6. Add the seasoned shrimp, and keep the heat on medium-low. Cook the shrimp for 3 minutes on each side until they turn pinkish.

7. Stir in the zest of lemon and the lemon juice. Add the prepared vegetables back to the pan. Stir to combine with the shrimp. Set aside.

8. In the steam spray. Cook the pasta following the company's specifications until attaining an al dente texture. Drain the pasta.

9. Transfer the cooked pasta in a large serving bowl and combine with the lemony-garlic shrimp and vegetables.

Nutrition: Calories: 474 Protein: 37 g Fat: 15 g Carbs: 46 g

DESSERT RECIPES

Cinnabon's Classic Cinnamon Rolls

Preparation Time: 2 Hours and 45 Minutes

Cooking Time: 15 Minutes

Servings: 12

Ingredients:

Dough:

- 1 cup warm milk (about 110 °F)
- 2 eggs
- 1/3 cup margarine, melted
- 4 ½ cups white bread flour
- 1 teaspoon salt
- ½ cup white sugar
- 2 ½ teaspoons rapid raising yeast
- 1 tablespoon all-purpose flour
- 1 cup brown sugar
- 2 ½ tablespoons cinnamon, ground
- 1/3 cup butter, softened

Frosting:

- 3 ounces cream cheese, softened

- ¼ cup butter, softened
- 1½ cups powdered sugar
- ½ teaspoon vanilla extract
- 1/8 teaspoon salt

Directions:

1. Arrange dough ingredients in bread machine pan following manufacturer's instructions. Select dough cycle and press Start.
2. Once the dough has reached double its original size, transfer onto surface lightly sprinkled with flour. Cover, and set aside for 10 minutes.
3. Preheat oven to 400 °F.
4. Mix brown sugar then cinnamon in a bowl.
5. Flatten dough into a rectangle, about 16 by 21 inches. Brush with 1/3 cup butter and sugar and cinnamon combination. Roll dough in a roll and cut it into 12 even pieces.
6. Handover slices onto a large baking sheet. Cover then let rest for 30 minutes or until size has doubled.
7. Bake for 15 minutes or pending lightly brown.
8. To make the frosting, combine all fixings in a bowl. Mix until smooth.
9. Remove rolls from oven and drizzle with frosting. Serve.

Nutrition: Calories 525, Total Fat 19 g, Carbs 82 g, Protein 9 g, Sodium 388 mg

Homemade Original Glazed Doughnuts from Krispy Kreme

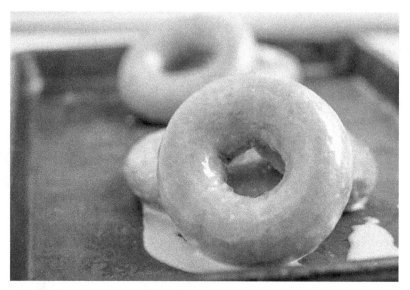

Preparation Time: 2 Hours

Cooking Time: 30 Minutes

Servings: 4

Ingredients:

- 2 packages of rapid raising yeast (¼ ounce each)
- ¼ cup warm water, about 105°F
- 1½ cup lukewarm milk, scalded then cooled
- ½ cup white sugar
- 1 teaspoon salt
- 2 eggs
- 1/3 cup shortening
- 5 cups all-purpose flour, then more for rolling dough

- Canola oil, for deep frying

Glaze:

- 1/3 cup butter, melted
- 2 cups powdered sugar
- 1½ teaspoon vanilla
- 3 tablespoons hot water

Directions:

1. In a bowl, melt yeast in water. Then, combine with milk, ½ cup sugar, salt, eggs, shortening, and 2 cups flour.

2. Using a mixer, whisk on low speed for 30 seconds while scraping sides of the bowl. On medium, continue to whisk for an additional 2 minutes. Mix in the rest of the flour until completely blended.

3. Let rest for about 50 minutes or until dough rises to twice its original size.

4. Transfer onto flat surface sprinkled with flour. Using a flour rolling pin, flatten dough until it is ½ inch thick. Cut into shape using a doughnut cutter. Let rest for another 30 minutes for the dough to rise.

5. In a deep fryer, preheat oil to 350°F.

6. Working in batches, carefully drop doughnuts into the deep fryer. Once floating, flip. Cook for approximately 1 minute per side or until lightly brown. Gently scoop out using a slotted spoon and transfer onto a plate lined with paper towels.

7. Mix all the glaze ingredients, except water, in a bowl until smooth and well-blended. Gradually add water, about 1 tablespoon at a time. Whisk until smooth.

8. Dip doughnuts in glaze. Serve.

Nutrition: Calories 303, Total Fat 11 g, Carbs 48 g, Protein 4 g, Sodium 161 mg

Mrs. Fields Snickerdoodle Cookies

Preparation Time: 50 Minutes

Cooking Time: 14 Minutes

Servings: 16 cookies

Ingredients:

- ½ cup butter, softened
- ½ cup granulated sugar
- 1/3 cup brown sugar
- 1 egg
- ½ teaspoon vanilla
- 1½ cups flour
- ¼ teaspoon salt
- ½ teaspoon baking soda
- ¼ teaspoon cream of tartar
- 2 tablespoons granulated sugar
- 1 teaspoon cinnamon

Directions:

1. Preheat oven to 300°F.
2. Using a mixer, combine softened butter and sugars. Mix in egg and vanilla. Combine until there are no longer lumps.
3. Mix flour, baking soda, salt, and cream of tartar in a bowl. Then, combine dry ingredients with wet ingredients. Blend well. Let rest in fridge for at least 30 minutes.

4. Mix 2 tablespoons granulated sugar and teaspoon of cinnamon together in a bowl.

5. Ball about 2½ tablespoons dough and coat evenly with cinnamon and sugar mixture. Transfer onto a baking sheet sprayed with cooking spray. Repeat for the rest of the dough.

6. Bake for no longer than 12 minutes. Cookies should be light golden brown but still soft, not crunchy.

7. Serve.

Nutrition: Calories 147, Total Fat 6 g, Carbs 22 g, Protein 2 g, Sodium 132 mg

DIY Pumpkin Scones from Starbucks

Preparation Time: 25 Minutes

Cooking Time: 15 Minutes

Servings: 8

Ingredients:

Scones:

- 2 cups all-purpose flour
- 1/3 cup brown sugar
- 1 teaspoon cinnamon
- 1 teaspoon baking powder
- ¾ teaspoon cloves, ground
- ½ teaspoon ginger, ground
- ½ teaspoon nutmeg, ground
- ½ teaspoon baking soda
- ¼ teaspoon salt
- ½ cup unsalted butter, cut into cubes (keep cold)
- ½ cup pumpkin puree
- 3 tablespoons milk
- 1 large egg
- 2 teaspoons vanilla extract
- Flour, for rolling dough

Glaze:

- 1 cup powdered sugar
- 2 tablespoons milk

Spiced glaze:

- 1 cup powdered sugar
- ¼ teaspoon cinnamon
- ¼ teaspoon cloves, ground
- ¼ teaspoon ginger, ground
- Pinch nutmeg
- 2 tablespoons milk

Directions:

1. Preheat oven to 400°F and fix a baking tray lined with parchment paper.
2. Mix flour, sugar, cinnamon, baking powder, cloves, ginger, nutmeg, baking soda, and salt in a bowl. Using your fingers, incorporate cold butter into the bowl until mixture is crumbly.
3. Stir together pumpkin puree, milk, egg, and vanilla in another bowl. Add to dry ingredients and mix until mixture becomes a soft dough.
4. Sprinkle a flat surface with flour. Transfer dough onto surface and knead for about 3 minutes. Flatten dough with a rolling pin into a large rectangle, about 1 inch thick and 10 by 7 inches. Cut in a cross to make 4 equal rectangles, then cut each rectangle diagonally. This makes 8 triangles.
5. Transfer dough onto baking tray, careful to keep triangles from touching. Bake for approximately 10 minutes or until baked through.

6. Prepare the glaze by mixing ingredients in a bowl until smooth. Do the same in a distinct bowl for the spiced glaze.

7. Allow scones to cool for about 10 minutes. Coat with glaze, then drip spiced glaze on top in zigzags.

8. Allow glazes to set before serving.

Nutrition: Calories 393, Total Fat 13 g, Carbs 64 g, Protein 5 g, Sodium 218 mg

Classic Cheesecake from The Cheesecake Factory

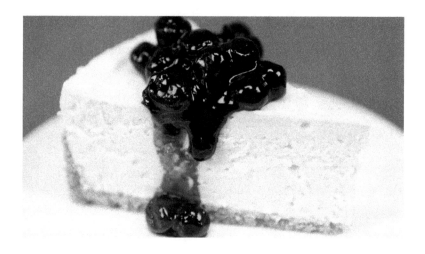

Preparation Time: 4 Hours and 15 Minutes

Cooking Time: 1 Hour and 5 Minutes

Servings: 12

Ingredients:

Crust:

- 1½ cups graham cracker crumbs
- ¼ teaspoon cinnamon, ground
- 1/3 cup margarine, melted

Filling:

- 4 8-ounce packages cream cheese, softened
- 1¼ cups white sugar
- ½ cup sour cream
- 2 teaspoons vanilla extract

- 5 large eggs

  Topping:

- ½ cup sour cream

- 2 teaspoons sugar

Directions:

1. Preheat oven to 475°F and heat a large skillet with ½ inch water inside.

2. Combine ingredients for the crust in a bowl. In a large pie pan lined with parchment paper, spread crust onto pan and press firmly. Cover with foil then keep in freezer until ready to use.

3. Combine ingredients for the filling, except for eggs, in a bowl. Scrape bowl while beating, until combination is smooth. Mix in eggs and beat until fully blended.

4. Take out crust from freezer and add filling onto crust, spreading evenly. Place pie pan into heated water bath (skillet in oven) and bake for about 12 minutes. Reduce heat to 350 °F. Continue to bake for about 50 minutes or until cake top is golden. Remove from oven and transfer skillet onto a wire rack to cool.

5. Prepare the topping by mixing all fixings in a bowl. Coat cake with topping, then cover. Keep inside refrigerator for at least 4 hours.

6. Serve cold.

Nutrition: Calories 519, Total Fat 39 g, Carbs 34 g, Protein 10 g,
Sodium 423 mg

Cracker Barrel's Double Fudge Coca Cola Chocolate Cake

Preparation Time: 20 Minutes

Cooking Time: 40 Minutes

Servings: 12

Ingredients:

Cake:

- Non-stick cooking spray
- ½ cup unsalted butter
- ½ cup vegetable oil
- 3 tablespoons unsweetened cocoa powder
- 1 cup Coca Cola™
- 2 cups all-purpose flour
- 2 cups granulated sugar
- ½ teaspoon salt
- 1 teaspoon baking soda
- ½ cup buttermilk
- 1 teaspoon pure vanilla extract
- 2 eggs

Frosting:

- ½ cup unsalted butter (1 stick), softened
- 1 teaspoon pure vanilla extract
- 3 tablespoons unsweetened cocoa powder
- 6 tablespoons Coca Cola™

- 4 cups powdered sugar

Directions:

1. Preheat oven to 350°F. Coat a large rectangular 9x13-inch baking pan with non-stick cooking spray.

2. Add the butter, oil, cocoa powder, and Coca Cola™ to a saucepan. Bring to a boil. Add mixture to the electric beater bowl. Add the flour, salt, sugar, and baking powder. Beat on medium speed until well combined.

3. Add one egg at a time. Add buttermilk and vanilla. Beat until well combined and cake batter is smooth.

4. Transfer prepared batter into pan, spreading evenly. Place in oven then bake for 40 minutes.

5. While the cake is in the oven, prepare the frosting. Using an electric beater, beat the butter into cream. Add 6 tablespoons of Coca Cola™, cocoa powder and vanilla. Beat until well combined.

6. Add the powdered sugar by increment of 1 cup at a time. Beat until frosting is smooth and fluffy.

7. Bring cake out of oven. While cake is still hot, spread the chocolate frosting evenly over the cake. Let cool down before covering with a plastic paper and place in the refrigerator until ready to serve. Serve with a scoop of vanilla ice cream, if wanted.

Nutrition: Calories 755, Total fat 25 g, Saturated fat 8 g, Carbs 108 g, Sugar 84 g, Fibers 2 g, Protein 5 g, Sodium 447 mg

CONCLUSION

The world is constantly changing, and the possibilities to eat out may change from one day to another.

This book reveals the secret recipes of America's most famous meals, and you can now create these delicious dishes at home, yourself. With the recipes in this book, you will be able to make your favorite restaurant or fast-food meals at home, making the whole family happy, while you save a lot of money. This copycat recipe book is a great gift for any occasion, and it will be appreciated by anyone who is eager to learn about the secrets of cooking delicious restaurant meals in the comfort of their own home. From now on, you will be able to enjoy the taste of famous dishes from your favorite restaurants and fast-food chains at home.

Family meals have always been a big deal at our house. There's just nothing quite like getting your friends and loved ones together in the dining room to enjoy a tasty, piping hot home cooked meal. I get that some folks love eating out, but for me, you just can't beat a home cooked meal when it comes to cost, health, and really the whole experience! But just like anyone else, I have my favorite foods that I enjoy time to time from restaurants.

My experiencing trying to create "copycat" recipes from restaurants began years ago in earnest when I attempted to replicate the Big Mac sauce my kids loved so much. Turns out there was a little more to it than just opening a bottle of Thousand Islands dressings.

I had fun creating these recipes and, hopefully, you have been able to choose one to create; for

me, all of them are tempting, so it's difficult to decide which one to make first. My strategy would be to pick one recipe for breakfast, one for lunch, one for a snack, and dinner every day. If you follow this recipe book and create the dishes described in it, your family will be amazed at your new cooking skills, and they will appreciate eating homemade food rather than always going to restaurants. I would like to thank you for investing your valuable time in reading my book; I am sure that it will be an easy-to-use and helpful tool in your kitchen.

You can entertain your friends and throw a house party with all the good meals from this book, but be careful because you might have them coming back often. My book of copycat recipes is not just for beginners, but also for experienced cooks who want to challenge themselves and have fun in the kitchen. I hope that you enjoy cooking these recipes, as well as eating them, and I wish you good appetite and a lot of fun!

If you have enjoyed this book, please leave me a review. For me, there is no greater reward than your satisfaction.

Leave me a comment if I miss any of your favorite restaurant's or brand's meals, so I can collect me

readers' favorites and create a Copycat Recipes part 2 for you soon.

CPSIA information can be obtained
at www.ICGtesting.com
Printed in the USA
BVHW052031120421
604748BV00001B/72

9 781801 830195